Basic Billing & Documentation for the Outpatient PMHNP

A nursing profession resource by
Lena Empyema

REFLECTS 2021 UPDATES TO CPT/HCPCS CODES & DOCUMENTATION REQUIREMENTS

BASIC BILLING & DOCUMENTATION

FOR THE OUTPATIENT

PMHNP

Answers to common questions asked by new
MENTAL HEALTH NURSE PRACTITIONERS & STUDENTS

LENA EMPYEMA

TABLE OF CONTENTS

TABLE OF CONTENTS

[1]

Introduction

One of the most common areas of frustration cited by new and student PMHNPs is the convoluted process of billing insurance payors for their services. Understandably, the system of numerically coding medical services with consideration to client-specific insurance coverage and guidelines that seem to change faster than evidence-based medicine takes some time to comprehend. However, for many PMHNPs expected to code and bill for their services as early as day one of employment, time to learn the craft of coding and billing is not a luxury at their disposal.

Medical coding and billing is its own specialty. Entire corporations exist for the purpose of providing this specific service to medical professionals. The concept of CPT coding alone has its own certification, and professionals in this field have entire careers revolving around coding and billing. This book is not meant to be a comprehensive resource on medical billing and coding. Rather, I wrote this book to bridge a gap between the specialty of medical coding and billing and the mental health care professionals who need to understand and apply the concepts to their clinical documentation. Further, knowing that there are PMHNPs who are responsible for coding and billing in addition to their clinical tasks, this book provides a foundation of the basics to apply in the clinical setting.

There are other resources in publication on the topic of coding and billing mental health care encounters, including the APA's own CPT code manual, which more than a thousand pages in length. Websites published by billing companies and Certified Professional Coders are also valuable tools to learn and properly utilize billing codes. A common theme among all of these resources, however, is the general textbook-like approach to defining various CPT and HCPCS codes, leaving the reader to decipher paragraphs of technical jargon and wondering how, *exactly*, to apply the information to their practice.

I noticed this deficit and created this resource to provide a more user-friendly experience in understanding, learning, and applying billing codes to PMHNP practice. With an educational background in Forensic Nursing focusing on the legalities of medical documentation, a professional background as a subject matter expert on documentation for nurses, and a history of multiple best-selling books on topics related to medical records, I wrote this book to provide real-world education on the topic of billing PMHNP services.

This book isn't written like a textbook. Some areas are written in first person, some in second person, and some in third person. I created visual graphs and drafted hypothetical examples throughout the book to appeal to professionals with any preferred style of learning. Because of this format, parts of the book may understandably be redundant to read cover-to-cover.

Inside this book, I provide an overview of coding mental health visits for billing purposes, discuss the most commonly-used CPT/HCPCS codes that PMHNPs across the U.S. use, explain a user-friendly algorithm that I created myself to help providers establish their own thought process for billing, and break down what criteria should be present in each note written to satisfy billing and coding requirements.

Because the real-world application of the concepts in this book go beyond educational narratives, I also created an online resource for PMHNP documentation which provides downloadable templates, custom data collection forms, and more graphic visuals, accessible from any phone or computer in the easy-to-navigate format of an e-course. It's all online for at www.PMHNPNotes.com.

To all PMHNPs, I hope this book makes your practice easier.

Lena Empyema
Lena Empyema, MSN

Disclaimer

The author of this book is not an attorney. This book should not be used as legal or medical advice. This book is not meant to assist with diagnoses, but rather to provide information about billing codes and corresponding documentation.

Leveraging Other Resources

The topics of billing, coding, and documentation are incredibly complex and dynamic. Like other areas of medicine, a working knowledge of the topic often means you have not memorized the entirety of the subject matter, but instead know where to reference more material as you need it.

This book should provide a basic knowledge of coding and billing for PMHNPs which will allow you to better understand and implement other resources available to you. It is purposefully written to be easy to reference.

If after reading this book, coding and billing still feels overwhelming alongside your other duties as a mental health care professional, know where to find other resources.

Outsourcing the majority of your billing to a third-party company is one way many professionals relieve the burden. Using a billing service to ensure that your services are billed to not only maximize the reimbursement for your services, but also maintain compliance with industry standards. Doing so will also allow you to focus your administrative efforts on comprehensive documentation. *I am not affiliated with any billing services, nor can I recommend one.*

[2]

Billing Codes &
Documentation:
Which comes first?

To fully grasp the concept of CPT and HCPCS codes, it is helpful to have a solid understanding of how to document clinical data in notes — but, to write complete and relevant notes, it is beneficial to have an understanding of the concepts of coding and billing. So, *is it the chicken or the egg?*

Like other aspects of clinical practice, it all goes hand-in-hand — and it will all come together.

One common area of confusion surrounds not just *how* to choose the right billing code, but *when*. Some clinics where PMHNPs practice provide just a few specialty services, which drastically limits the number of codes those professionals have to know. In other areas of practice, the mental health services provided may be more open-ended. In any of these cases, for providers new to assigning billing codes and ensuring adequate documentation, the real-world process can be overwhelming.

The answer to what to do *first* starts before you first meet the client. When a visit is scheduled, it should be somewhat clear that the encounter will fit into one of three main categories: a new client intake, a medical service for an established client, or a non-medical therapy service for an established client. These broad categories are discussed more in-depth later in the book.

Knowing which general category any given client visit best fits, you as the provider can structure your interaction around the type of visit. For example, an initial visit with a new client should include more in-depth assessment and history questions, whereas a follow-up on the efficacy of a new prescription can safely be abbreviated to a focused assessment.

The data you collect during the encounter provide the contents for your notes. Not every piece of information you learn or collect during the interaction will be pertinent enough to document, nor pertinent to pinpointing a billing code. Later in the book, I will discuss specifics of documentation to include in your notes, as well as tips for excluding extraneous data to streamline your charting process. The pertinent highlights of the encounter should be documented clearly but succinctly, and then used to determine exactly which service you ended up providing. The definitions for each five-digit billing code are detailed and specific. When the encounter has ended and you have a clear picture of exactly what you ended up doing for the client, you can choose the code that best reflects what was done, to include a primary code and any applicable add-on codes (some visits may have no add-on codes, others may have one or two).

To summarize, the clinical process generally follows the pattern of choosing a broad category, documenting pertinent highlights in a note, then using those data points to choose a specific code within the broad category that you chose initially.

Example

Let's use 90832 as an example (the code for a 30-minute psychotherapy session).

In this hypothetical example, your employer states that your objective as a new PMHNP is to schedule 14 clients per day and bill each of them 90832.

You can approach each session with the template for a 90832 session as your prompt to structure the encounter. For some clients, the encounter may proceed exactly as structured. You can capture data specific to a 30-minute psychotherapy session, document accordingly, perform no additional interventions, and appropriately bill such visits as 90832 with no add-on services.

If, during the session, the plan changes, you may need to reevaluate which code best fits the services that you end up providing. If, for example, the client arrives at a scheduled talk therapy appointment and reports new symptoms, an E/M code for an established client may become more accurate as a primary billing code as you evaluate the change in your client's status and consider possible diagnostics, labs, or medication changes. If psychotherapy still occurs after the medical evaluation, an add-on time-based psychotherapy code can then be billed in addition to the E/M code.

This ability to change the course of action from a therapy-centered visit to a medical-centered appointment is relatively unique to the PMHNP. Other mental health care professionals such as psychologists and counselors may more frequently schedule and provide psychotherapy sessions, and if the client brings up a medical concern during the therapy visit, those licensed professionals with different scopes of practice would not be able to pivot to a medical-based billing code. Thus, the versatility of a PMHNP license can create additional confusion when choosing a billing code. Still, knowing and understanding the basics of coding specific to your license can help you establish a quick and accurate thought process.

[3]

Basics of Coding for Mental Health Care

Codes on Codes on Codes:

Applying the concepts of coding and billing to your practice starts with understanding and differentiating types of codes used, including:

- ICD-10
- CPT
- HCPCS
- RVUs

Acronyms to know

CMS: Center for Medicare & Medicaid Services
ICD: International Classification of Disease
HCPCS: Healthcare Common Procedure Coding System
E/M: Evaluation and Management
CPT: Current Procedural Terminology
AMA: American Medical Association

Types of Codes

There are multiple coding systems that impact documentation in your practice. Each of them essentially serves to translate medical information into a number with a specific definition that non-medical personnel can understand.

One set of codes commonly used by PMHNPs is the ICD-10 code system to assign each diagnosis a numerical code. Another is the CPT code system which translates services rendered into numerical codes that insurance companies can use to process claims. Yet another code system is HCPCS, which also translate medical services into numerical codes used by insurance companies to process claims, yet carry some distinct differences from CPT codes, which will be broken down in the next few sections.

ICD-10

There are two types of ICD-10 codes to include ICD-10-**CM** and ICD-10-**PCS.**

ICD-10-CM codes correspond to the reason the client is seeking care. These are for outpatient claims and are the more common of the codes used for reimbursement of psychiatric and mental health claims.

ICD-10-PCS are for inpatient procedures. They are used to determine Medicare Severity-Diagnosis Groups.

HCPCS

HCPCS stands for Healthcare Common Procedure Coding System. Rather than pronouncing each of the five letters as an acronym, many providers refer to these codes aloud as "hick-picks."

HCPCS are billing codes used to process insurance claims for services rendered to a patient. The Centers for Medicare and Medicaid developed the HCPCS system to make the codes available to the public. There are three levels of HCPCS coding. Level I HCPCS codes mirror CPT codes. The five-digit HCPCS codes for Level I are the same as the corresponding five-digit code for CPT. However, HCPCS is specific to Medicare and Medicaid. So, if you choose a five-digit code to bill a client service, such as 90832 for a psychotherapy session, if you are billing Medicare or Medicaid for that session, that five-digit number is now a HCPCS code. If you are billing an insurance provider other than Medicare or Medicaid with the same number, it is a CPT code.

While CPT codes and HCPCS codes are not *entirely* interchangeable, the terms are often used interchangeably to discuss billing Medicare and Medicaid. When in doubt, referring to a code as a "billing code" should be easily understood by all pertinent professionals in the industry.

CPT

CPT® **codes** are copyright by the American Medical Association. Providers pay an annual fee to the AMA to gain access to CPT codes and use them for billing purposes.

CPT stands for Current Procedural Terminology. These codes, like HCPCS, are a way to translate medical services into a specific five-digit number easily understood by insurance companies to process claims. There are thousands of CPT codes used in the U.S., though a much smaller number apply to mental health clients.

RVUs

RVU stands for relative value unit. This number is as part of a multi-step formula to determine the amount of money a provider will be reimbursed for any given billing code. This formula is computerized and there is no real reason to evaluate it in-depth other than to understand that the definition of an RVU is complex and dynamic across the country.

In broad terms, the formula uses three types of RVUs (work RVUs, practice expense RVUs, and malpractice RVUs), factors in the cost of performing medical services in the specific geographical location where the services are being billed (Geographic Practice Cost Index), then is multiplied by the Medicare conversion factor, which is a different number every year.

An excellent free tool to help visualize the differences in RVUs among codes is the Medicare Physician Fee Schedule. This online tool allows you to input a billing code and calculate the current repayment formula based on current values. Because the tool is the property of CMS, the codes are referred to as HCPCS. Recall that Level I HCPCS codes equate to CPT codes when applied to Medicare and Medicaid clients.

The calculator is available at www.cms.gov/medicare/physician-fee-schedule/search.

The 35-page PDF explaining how to use the calculator is available at www.cms.gov/files/document/2020-physician-fee-schedule-guide.pdf.

"Should I choose billing codes based on the number of RVUs they are worth?"

The most accurate yet inherently vague answer to this question is that billing codes should be assigned to client encounters based on which code most accurately reflects the services rendered.

RVUs and total reimbursement for services rendered is important for providers. Some providers even have a salary structure based on total RVUs rendered to clients over the course of a year. Others receive bonuses based on RVUs. (If you are not a professional receiving bonuses or pay based on this productivity model, your new level of understanding of how your services generate money for a clinic could be useful in negotiating one).

For instances in which one of two codes could be accurate (such as codes 99205 and 90792 for a new client intake), the *first* factor to consider is not which of the two codes has a higher number of RVUs assigned to it, but whether the client's insurance coverage will reimburse for both codes. If the client is only eligible for one of the two codes, then the answer is easy: the code which will result in a successful insurance claim should be used.

If the client has coverage for either of the two codes in this example, and the encounter itself can justify either 90792 or 99205, then it is appropriate to consider RVUs.

Just like other concepts in coding and billing, there is not a one-size-fits-all answer to every possible scenario. Rather, you should apply the information in this book to *your* clients at *your specific* place of employment.

Overview of Billing Codes

Definitions to know

New patient: For billing purposes, this is an individual not seen by you or another provider in the same specialty and working in the same medical group as you within the past 3 years.

Established patient: For billing purposes, any individual who has been seen by you or another provider in the same specialty and working in the same medical group as you within the past 3 years.

"What purpose do billing codes Serve?"

Billing codes serve to translate medical services into one or more five-digit numbers that can be easily understood by insurance companies to calculate claim reimbursements. Use of standardized codes creates uniformity for similar services among providers nationwide, and places those medical services in a format that non-medical professionals can understand and analyze to calculate insurance reimbursement.

"What do I do with them?"

Ultimately, you will use billing codes to submit claims to insurance companies to generate revenue for services rendered.

After providing services to your clients, you will select the billing code that best describes the work you performed and fill out a form called CMS-1500. The insurance company will process form CMS-1500 and use the codes you provided to calculate reimbursement rates for your clients.

Categories of Billing Codes

There are thousands of billing codes that can apply to medical appointments. Specific to mental health care, the pool of potential CPT codes is smaller, but still significant.

If you have started diving into the topic of billing codes, you may have realized quickly that selecting a single code can vary based on the client's insurance payor, the state you practice in, the client's recent track record of medical visits, and other minute details.

Fortunately, like other daunting areas of medicine, there is a systemic and predictable algorithm that can help you determine the best billing code for most encounters, which is based upon *what you did for the client and how long it took you to do it.*

Further, when this algorithm doesn't seem to work for you or you find yourself spending more time talking to insurance payors than clients, there are a range of professional billing services available.

I am not affiliated with any medical billing service, nor can I provide a recommendation for a service to use.

The major categories of codes that PMHNPs use include the following. **The three most common categories that PMHNPs use are bolded.**

1. **Psychiatric diagnostic evaluations**

2. **Evaluation and management services (E/M)**

3. **Individual psychotherapy**

4. Family therapy

5. Group therapy

6. Therapy for crisis

Within each of these categories, there are multiple difference codes further specifying the exact services rendered, and how long was spent caring for the client. For example, within the category of E/M billing codes, there are separate codes for *inpatient* care versus *outpatient* care. The category of *outpatient E/M codes* is then further broken down into four possible codes for new clients and five codes for established clients.

Many client encounters may be easily summarized with a single billing code. For those that aren't, there are nearly as many add-on codes to assist in capturing the entirety of a visit. For example, continuing with the first example of 90832 (individual psychotherapy lasting 30 minutes), a common add-on code is 90785 for interactive complexity, such as a therapy session for an adolescent who is not forthcoming with contributions. (There is a long list of situations that warrant the use of add-on 90785, so this is just one example).

The three most common categories of codes that apply to PMHNP visits will be discussed in more detail.

1. Psychiatric Diagnostic Evaluation
2. Evaluation and Management (E/M)
3. Individual Psychotherapy

1. Evaluation and Management

Abbreviated E/M, evaluation and management codes are general codes that physicians and non-physician providers in *all* areas of medicine use. In total, there are thousands of E/M codes that refer to all modalities of medicine, but only a few specific to mental health care.

Because they are not specific to mental health, their definitions are related generally to medical services rendered. All E/M codes are five digits in length and start with "99."

E/M codes are among the most common codes that apply to psychiatric client encounters for a few reasons.

First, there are 9 potential E/M codes to apply to mental health visits. They are categorized in ascending level of complexity and, as of 2021, have **time ranges** assigned to each to help providers objectively choose a code. (See next section for why this is an important update).

Four of these E/M codes apply only to "new" clients (which doesn't always mean a client who is just new to *you* – see the definition a few pages back) and five of them are just for "established" clients.

For PMHNPs, E/M codes are used to bill visits that are more medically oriented than strictly psychotherapy or psychiatric evaluation. This designation is important, because PMHNPs have the scope of practice to perform medical services for mental health clients (such as prescription, laboratory work, or diagnostic services) which not all types of licensed mental health providers can offer.

As of 2021, E/M Codes are Easier to Select

In 2021, the outpatient E/M billing codes underwent changes to their leveling system which made it significantly faster and easier for providers to choose the correct E/M code.

Understanding an overview of the previous, more complex method of choosing the right E/M code is of potential pertinence because a huge number of resources are still published and available online which discuss the old system, which could create confusion.

In previous years, *time* was not the deciding factor to use a certain E/M code. Rather, an analysis of three components was necessary to determine *the complexity of medical-decision making* (commonly abbreviated MDM) a provider used for any given E/M encounter. The correct code was assigned according to four potential levels of complexity.

The new definitions for selecting E/M codes still allows providers to choose a code based on the complexity of medical decision-making, if they prefer to do so rather than choosing based on time spent rendering care. However, the instances when this would be necessary are very rare. Theoretically, if a provider rendered services to a very complex client which required a high level of medical decision-making but the provider spent only a short amount of time rendering that care, it could be more beneficial to choose a higher code which, in this specific example, may only be justified by citing the complexity of medical decision-making.

In the vast majority of cases, however, as the complexity of a client case increases, the time spent directly rendering care and indirectly coordinating services for that client will also increase. Thus, most of the time, a higher E/M code can be fairly justified by the total time spent providing care for a client. Less complex clients will require less time from the provider.

The added benefit to choosing E/M codes based on time rather than the medical decision-making algorithm is that it is quite simple to objectively justify a time-based code by clearly stating in the clinical documentation the **total number of minutes spent** providing care for a certain client. In the event of an audit, the ability to numerically prove that a certain E/M code was properly billed to the insurance payor is much easier to do than walking through a multi-step algorithm which historically resulted in subjective differences among billing providers. For example, under the previous MDM model, one provider may apply the MDM algorithm to a case and determine that he or she used a moderate amount of medical decision-making, while another provider could apply the algorithm to a clinically similar case and conclude that he or she used a high level of MDM.

The definition of **time spent providing care** for the client also updated as of 2021. Whereas previous stipulations required that more than 50 percent of the time be spent in face-to-face counseling, the totality of time now constitutes any time spent coordinating care, communicating with third parties related to client problems, scheduling follow-ups, and reviewing medical records or lab results in addition to face-t0-face time spent counseling the client.

With these changes, there theoretically is no longer a need to spend time evaluating the minutiae of data collected for its relevance in the medical decision-making process. All outpatient E/M codes can now be chosen based on how much time was spent caring for the client.

Previous resources used dozens of pages of text and charts to explain the MDM algorithm -- for the sake of brevity and clarity, I am not going to elaborate further on the algorithm itself.

Until or unless there is an update which again transforms the way providers choose outpatient E/M codes, providers can simply tally the total number of minutes spent to choose the correct code from the relevant category.

Considerations When Choosing an E/M Code

Is the client inpatient or outpatient?

As aforementioned, there are nine E/M codes which can apply to outpatient PMHNP clients. For inpatient care, there is a different set. This resource discusses only the outpatient codes.

Of note, in years prior, there were also different codes for clients receiving care in an office versus a hospital. Now, there is no differentiation in CPT/HCPCS codes based where care was rendered, just differences in outpatient care versus inpatient care.

On the official form used for billing insurance companies (called CMS-1500), there is, however, still a place to designate *place of service* using a two-digit code which is different from a billing code. I will discuss CMS-1500 in much more detail in a later section.

Is the client new to your practice, or established?

Clients **new to your practice group** must not have met with you or any other providing practicing the same specialty as you and working within your medical group within the past 3 years.

New clients receiving an E/M service can be billed with one of four codes:

- 99202 for 15-29 minutes
- 99203 for 30-44 minutes
- 99204 for 45-59 minutes
- 99205 for 60-74 minutes

Established clients have met with your or another provider in your medical group working in the same specialty as you at some point in the last three years.

Established outpatient clients receiving an E/M service can be billed with one of five codes:

- 99211 (fewer than 10 minutes)

- 99212 for 10-19 minutes
- 99213 for 20-29 minutes
- 99214 for 30-39 minutes
- 99215 for 40-54 minutes

2. Psychiatric Diagnostic Evaluation

Codes 90791 and 90792 are used for psychiatric diagnostic evaluations. They are very similar, with the only difference being that 90791 is for the diagnostic evaluation of a client not receiving medical services, whereas 90792 includes medical services rendered to a client.

Because medical services are within the scope of practice for PMHNPs, 90792 should easily be justified. Code 90791 is used by professionals whose scope of practice does not include medical services.

What constitutes a "medical service" (thereby justifying code 90792 instead of 90791?

While there is not a comprehensive list of the services that qualify as "medical" for the purpose of justifying 90792 over 90791, the answer comes down to the PMHNP's scope of practice. PMHNP responsibilities include medication prescription, ordering lab tests, and performing physical assessments, all skills which counselors and non-medical therapists cannot render. Differentiating between 90791 and

90792 is easily done by comparing your scope of practice to the more limited scope of practice that another type of licensed mental health professional cannot provide.

- o Writing a prescription
- o Recommending a prescription
- o Performing a physical exam
- o Modifying psychiatric treatment to accommodate medical comorbidities

For a new client, why would a 90792 code be used instead of a higher level "new client" E/M code?

90792 and, as an example, 99205, are both used for the initial diagnosis of a new client, or for diagnosing a new behavioral health concern. Most commonly, the psychiatric diagnostic evaluations are used for the initial intake for a new client.

Reimbursement can vary among insurance payors, but most policies only provide coverage for a psychiatric diagnostic evaluation code to be used one time per year, per client. Some insurance payors allow a psychiatric diagnostic evaluation to be billed every six months. The reason for a second psychiatric diagnostic evaluation would be the onset of new symptoms or changes in the client's status which could indicate a new psychiatric diagnosis.

For most insurance payors, prior authorization to use either diagnostic evaluation code is not required. Independently performing eligibility and benefits verification for clients will help determine if their individual policy covers 90791 or 90792 as well as other important information for billing purposes.

Billing a diagnostic evaluation code is reimbursed at a higher rate than individual psychotherapy sessions, so it is beneficial to bill as 90792 rather than an E/M code when applicable to your client's initial visit.

90792 is equated with more RVUs than an E/M code, and thus are reimbursed at a higher rate than an E/M visit. It is used when medical services are included as part of a psychiatric diagnostic evaluation. Because medical services are part of the client encounter, a standard psychotherapy visit can be ruled out, leaving the only other comparable option as an outpatient E/M code.

That being said, it is not wrong to use an E/M code instead of code 90792. Doing so is not fraudulent nor should it raise any flags to potential auditors. In most cases, it is simply billed at a slightly lower rate than code 90792.

Specifics to know about code 90792:

- This code cannot be billed to a client on the same day that an E/M service is billed to the client by the same provider
- Sessions must last at least 16 minutes and can last as long as 90 minutes. Most psychiatric diagnostic evaluation sessions last about 60 minutes, but time is not a factor in choosing this code.

Interview components of a typical 90792 session:

- o Complete medical history
- o Complete psychiatric history
- o Mental status examination
- o Evaluation of the client's ability to respond to treatment
- o Initial plan of treatment

Documentation for a 90792 exam should include:

- Total time spent providing care for client (to ensure that at least 16 minutes elapsed, and to justify potential use of an add-on code for extended time if the session lasts more than 90 minutes)
- Modality of chosen treatment
- Suggested frequency of treatment
- DSM-5 diagnosis
- Client's symptoms
- Client's functional status
- Focused mental status examination
- Prognosis
- Proposed treatment plan

3. Individual Psychotherapy

A psychotherapy session should be coded with no medical services were performed which could warrant billing an E/M session.

Recall that if you provide a medical service in addition to psychotherapy, you can bill the client for an E/M service, the use an add-on code to include psychotherapy. Both the E/M code and the psychotherapy codes are time-based. During the encounter, you should track the amount of time spent providing the E/M service. The clock should start over when the psychotherapy session begins. Bill the E/M service based on the amount of time spent providing evaluation or management services, then use the add-on code which corresponds to the correct time range to bill for the psychotherapy session.

Documentation for a psychotherapy encounter should include:

- Total time spent in session
- Reason for encounter
- DSM-5 diagnosis
- Themes of topics discussed
- Risk assessment
- Interventions used
- Progress towards goals
- Any updates to treatment plan
- Expected outcomes with continued adherence to treatments

Primary psychotherapy codes include:

- 90832 for 30 minutes (range is 16-37 minutes).
- 90834 for 45 minutes (range is 38-52 minutes).
- 90837 for 60 minutes (53+ minutes).
-

When billing for a primary E/M encounter with add-on psychotherapy following, the add-oncodes for the psychotherapy component are:

- 90833 for 30 minutes (range is 16-37 minutes).
- 90836 for 45 minutes (range is 38-52 minutes).
- 90838 for 60 minutes (53+ minutes).

[4]

How to Assign a Billing Code for Each Encounter

The legal and monetary implications of this administrative task make it a daunting one. Even if outsourcing billing to a third party, the individual clinician is still responsible for ensuring that the most accurate and appropriate CPT codes are used for their services.

The information in this chapter should help you establish your own though process for assigning a billing code to each encounter.

Tips to Begin Mastering Billing Code Selection in Your Practice

With coding systems as complex as CPT and HCPCS, mastery takes time. While you work through the book and apply concepts to your practice, consider these four tips for streamlining your learning process.

- o Start and maintain a list of the billing codes you use most frequently. A good place to start is with the PMHNP Coding Algorithm I created, which you will find later in this chapter. A larger version is available free for viewing at **www.pmhnpnotes.com**.

- o Do not try to memorize all the CPT codes you could potentially use. Not only do these codes change every few years, but identifying the correct code is a quick process online once you understand the general concept of billing codes.

- o Write notes from templates to ensure that you are meeting all documentation requirements before submitting a claim to an insurance payor.

- o Before submitting a claim, ensure that the client's eligibility and benefits cover the billing code you want to use. In some offices, the task of contacting insurance companies to discuss client coverage may fall on the PMHNP. If you use a billing service, eligibility confirmation is generally included.

Time-Based Codes:
What counts towards billable time?

- Preparing to see the client by reviewing tests and records
- Obtaining and/or reviewing the client's history from another provider or facility
- Interpreting test or lab results and communicating the findings to the client and, if applicable, family
- Performing an exam or evaluation
- Providing counseling and education to the client and, if applicable, client's family
- Coordinating care

As You Read, Consider:
3 Most Common Reasons for Claim Denials

1. **Client's insurance does not provide coverage for the billing code submitted.**

Not all insurance payors provide coverage for all billing codes. Some allow a certain code to be billed a limited number of times per year. Even when a CPT or HCPCS accurately reflects the services rendered, there is no guarantee that it is eligible for payment by the client's insurance policy. Thus, verifying the client's benefits before submitting a claim is an important step. This is a task that can be outsourced to administrative personnel at your place of employment, your billing department, or a third-party billing company. If none of these options are available to you, then contacting insurance companies to verify benefits will fall to you.

2. **Incorrect CPT or HCPCS codes.**

Choosing the wrong billing code for services rendered will result in a claim denial by the insurance provider. This can include using outdated codes that may have worked in the past, but are now replaced by a different code. Billing codes do not change weekly or monthly, but as often as every year or two, the codes that you use the most often may change. Ensuring you are up-to-date on the most current set of billing codes is important. Of pertinence, this book was published in

2022 based on the most recent updates that were made in 2021.

Choosing the wrong code can mean leaving money on the table, or, worse, can constitute fraud. It is vitally important to understand which codes to choose for your clients and how to document to support the codes that you billed.

For PMHNPs, coding is the process of translating the services rendered to a client into one or more existing codes which insurance companies use to process claims.

Every client encounter is translated into at least one code. Many codes include a bundle of services so that even when the provider performs more than one service or intervention, a single code can still capture the entirety of a visit. When a single code cannot capture every service that a client received during an encounter, add-on codes can be billed in addition to the primary code.

Mistakes in coding include undercoding, upcoding, and unbundling.

Undercoding occurs when the billing code applied to a client encounter correlates to a lower amount of reimbursement. Undercoding can occur unintentionally, such as when a provider is not certain that the data or documentation supports a higher level of billing. However, it is not uncommon for providers to intentionally under-code a service to assist the client in saving money, or in hopes of avoiding an audit. No matter the intentionality or specific reason for undercoding, it is by definition a fraudulent offense.

On the opposite end of the spectrum is **upcoding**, when a provider assigns a billing code that correlates to an amount of reimbursement in excess of what should be billed. Upcoding is also fraudulent. Unintentional upcoding can be avoided by ensuring that the data in your documentation is on par with the requirements of the code that you assign to a client encounter.

Unbundling is the cumbersome process of assigning individual billing codes to each unique service rendered to a client rather than choosing a single billing code that captures the entirety of a visit. Historically, providers have unbundled billing codes in hopes of being reimbursed more money than they would receive if a visit was billed under a single, all-inclusive code. Other resources have compared hypothetical reimbursement rates for using a single code versus using three or four unbundled codes, and found a remarkably similar rate of reimbursement. With no monetary reason to unbundle billing codes, PMHNPs should avoid the time-consuming process of unbundling and instead choose as few codes as can accurately reflect the level and length of services provided to a client.

3. **Inaccurate time-based codes**.

One of the most common "wrong code" errors is submitting a time-based code (psychotherapy and the newest E/M codes as of 2021) for the wrong amount of time spent rendering care. Ensure that the total number of minutes you spent providing services to a client is prominently documented in your notes, and ensure that the code you select reflects the correct amount of time.

Quick-Reference Codes for PMHNPs

While aforementioned and explained in more detail in previous sections, this section lists the most-used codes along with a brief description for quicker reference during future look-ups.

These billing codes can change regularly and this text may not be the most up-to-date version of billing codes, nor is this book written to be a comprehensive resource for understanding billing codes in psychiatric care. The CPT manual published by the APA is in excess of 1,200 pages long! That manual is the best and most comprehensive source of information for billing codes. As I wrote this book about charting and documentation practices, I discuss billing codes for the purpose of understanding how to satisfactorily document to meet the requirements of certain codes and categories of codes.

PSYCHIATRIC DIAGNOSTIC EVALUATION

90792 | Psychiatric diagnosis interview and examination (PDE) *with medical services*. This code can be used only one time per client at the outset of the illness and must meet specific criteria:

- Medication prescription

- Coordination of medication management
- Order or reviewing medical diagnostic studies

EVALUATION & MANGEMENT OF NEW CLIENTS

By definition, a new client must be someone who has not received any medical services any provider in your group practice who practices the same specialty as the one that you practice.

99202 | New outpatient with straightforward decision making, 15-29 minutes.

99203 | New outpatient with straightforward decision making, 30-44 minutes.

99204 | New outpatient with straightforward decision making, 45-59 minutes.

99205 | High complexity problems addressed.

EVALUATION & MANGEMENT OF ESTABLISHED CLIENTS

99211 | Established patient with minimal problems not requiring the physical presence of a licensed professional (such as a nurse visit to answer a client's question).

99212 | Established patient, stable, 10-19 minutes.

99213 | Established patient, 20-29 minutes.

99214 | Established patient, 30-39 minutes.

99215 | Established patient, 30-54 minutes. High complexity problems addressed.

INDIVIDUAL PSYCHOTHERAPY

90832 | Individual psychotherapy session, 16-37 minutes.

90834 | Individual psychotherapy session, 38-52 minutes.

90837 | Individual psychotherapy session, 53 minutes or longer.

FAMILY & GROUP PSYCHOTHERAPY

Specific to Medicare billing, psychotherapy for a single family is more likely to be approved than therapy for multiple families on the basis that multi-family therapy cannot be tailored to meet a specific client's medical needs.

90846, 90847 | Family psychotherapy, 26 minutes or longer.

90849 | multi-family group psychotherapy.

90853 | Group psychotherapy.

EMERGENCY SESSIONS/CRISIS INTERVENTION

For clients in great distress requiring immediate attention or for clients who are experiencing a life-threatening situation.

For crisis sessions that last fewer than 30 minutes, use a code for a regular psychotherapy appointment.

90839 | First 60 minutes of psychotherapy for crisis

90840 | Add-on code for **each additional 30 minutes** of psychotherapy for crisis

99050 | Add-on code for services **provided after hours (when clinic is usually closed).**

99051 | Add-on code for services provided during regularly scheduled hours on evenings, weekends, or holidays.

Other Common Add-on Codes:

E/M plus Psychotherapy

If the basis of your visit is medication management, such as a follow-up about a new prescription, your primary billing code will be an E/M code. If you then provide talk therapy after addressing medical-related concerns, the code for psychotherapy then becomes an add-on code to the primary E/M code.

Just as a standalone psychotherapy session is billed according to time, so are the add-on codes for psychotherapy following an E/M encounter.

These add-ons are as follows:

90833 | 30 minutes of psychotherapy with E/M service

90836 | 45 minutes of psychotherapy with E/M service

90838 | 60 minutes of psychotherapy with E/M service

Interactive Complexity

90785 | Interactive complexity

Interactive complexity refers to barriers in communication that increase the workload for the provider. It is most commonly used for visits with pediatric clients, but there are a few instances during interactions with adults when 90785 is also warranted:

1. Maladaptive communication skills which affects the ability of the provider to interact with the client, such as:
   a. Clients with high anxiety
   b. Clients with high reactivity
   c. Providers having to ask a question repeatedly to elicit a response
2. Emotional or behavioral conditions inhibiting the implementation of a treatment plan
3. When circumstances during a visit create a "mandated report" situation in which the provider will spend time reporting findings to the appropriate agency (such as in abuse or neglect cases).
4. Use of play equipment or special devices to help client contribute thoughts, feelings, and reactions to sessions.

When can 90785 <u>not</u> be applied?

When the only barrier to communication is that the client speaks a language different from the primary language spoken by the provide and thus requires the assistance of an interpreter or translator, 90785 cannot be applied. Charging an additional code to clients who speak a different language is a discrimination issue.

If the client happens to speak a different language than the provider *and* one of the above situations occurs, 90785 can be safely applied.

May be reported, as appropriate, with 90791, 90792, 90832, 90833, 90834, 90836, 90853, 90837, and 99202-99215.

Decision-Making Algorithm for PMHNPs New to Billing Codes

Determining the most appropriate billing code(s) for a client encounter is a systematic yet complex process. Learning and understanding the basics of this process discusses in previous sections is the first step to being able to apply this algorithm to your practice.

To help the puzzle pieces of knowledge begin to fit together, I created this seven-step system to break down selecting the most common CPT billing codes used by PMHNPs.

"Reading these seven steps is still confusing for me. How can I better understand it?"

Rather than reading this process from start to finish, instead consider a recent client encounter, and follow the steps as if you are using them to choose a billing code for a real case. Doing so is less confusing than attempting to read start to finish and retain the procedure.

Also, review the graphic I created to visualize the process. As a reminder, this is a consolidated algorithm addressing only the most common reasons for visits and most common billing codes used. The graphic is not comprehensive (because it wouldn't fit on a single page!) but demonstrates how to apply the thought process to select the most appropriate billing code.

"When does this decision-making algorithm *not* apply?"

This seven-step process is not all-inclusive. Rather, it addresses the most common codes PMHNPs use to bill their client encounters. Recall that there are thousands of CPT codes, so covering each possible billing scenario succinctly is not possible. If you possess special certifications or work in a specialty area, you may not use these common codes as frequently as other PMHNPs in more standard outpatient positions.

Further, there are many options for add-on codes not included in this process. Add-on codes can vary widely based on client demographics and individual situations. A few of the most common add-on codes are addressed in this seven-step process, but there are many more that may be available to you.

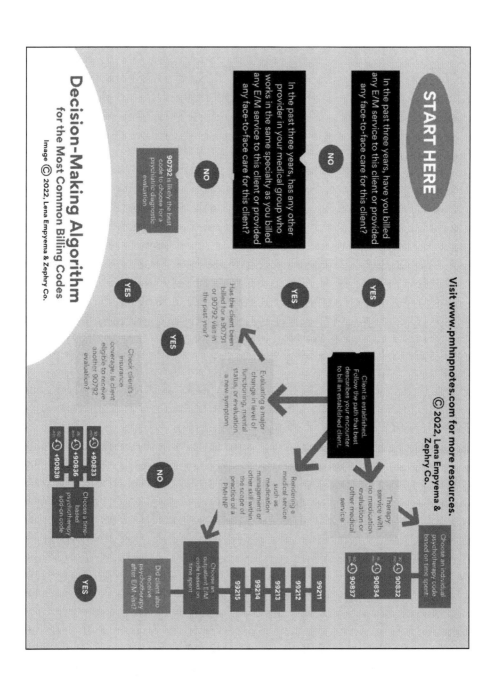

START HERE

Visit www.pmhnpnotes.com for more resources.
© 2022, Lena Empyema & Zephry Co.

In the past three years, have you billed any E/M service to this client or provided any face-to-face care for this client?

NO → In the past three years, has any other provider in your medical group who works in the same specialty as you billed any E/M service to this client or provided any face-to-face care for this client?

NO → 90792 is likely the best code to choose for a psychiatric diagnostic evaluation

YES → Client is established. Follow the path that best describes your encounter to bill an established client.

YES → Evaluating a major change in level of functioning, mental status, or evaluation a new symptom.

Has the client been billed for a 90791 or 90792 visit in the past year?

YES → Check client's insurance coverage. Is client eligible to receive another 90792 evaluation?

YES → Choose a time-based psychotherapy add-on code
+90833
+90836
+90838

Rendering a medical service such as medication management or other skill within the scope of a practice of a PMHNP.

NO → Choose an outpatient E/M code based on time spent.
99211
99212
99213
99214
99215

Did client also receive psychotherapy after E/M visit?

YES →

Therapy service with no medication evaluation or other medical service

Choose an individual psychotherapy code based on time spent.
90832
90834
90837

Decision-Making Algorithm
for the Most Common Billing Codes
Image © 2022, Lena Empyema & Zephry Co.

52

CONSIDER ANY CLIENT ENCOUNTER AND START WITH STEP 1:

1. Have you billed any E/M service or provided face-to-face care for this client in the past three years?
    a. If no, proceed to next question.
    b. If yes, proceed to Question #4.
2. Has another provider in your medical group who works in the same specialty as you billed any E/M service or provided face-to-face care for this client in the past three years?
    a. If no, proceed to next question.
    b. If yes, proceed to Question #4.
3. "NO" to Questions 1 & 2 means the client is **new**. Your first encounter will be an intake during which time you assess the client. There is more than one code available for a new client intake. In most cases, **90792** is the correct choice, **unless:**
    a. **Possible exception #1:** You experience a rare instance in which you perform a psychiatric diagnostic evaluation and provide no medical services, in which case, 90791 is more appropriate. This is rare because the PMHNP scope of practice includes applicable medical services, so billing for 90791 is below the scope of practice of a PMHNP.

b. Possible exception #2: You **must** also bill for psychotherapy on the same day. In this case, select an E/M code specifically for new clients (time-based as of 2021) and use the corresponding time-based psychotherapy add-on code, because psychotherapy cannot be billed on the same day as a psychiatric diagnostic evaluation.

c. Possible exception #3: The client has an insurance plan which does not provide coverage for billing 90792. Of note, 90792 is covered for most clients with Medicare, Medicaid, and other major insurers.

4. "YES" to either Question #1 or Question #2 means the client is **established**. Choosing a code is based on what services you are providing this client today, and how long you spend providing them.

    a. If you are rendering psychotherapy with no medication management, proceed to Question #5.

    b. If you are providing medication management services, proceed to Question #6.

    c. If you are assessing a major change in the client's level of functioning, mental status, or the onset of a new symptoms, proceed to Question #7.

5. Psychotherapy codes for established clients are time-based.

    a. If you spent 16-37 minutes providing psychotherapy, use code **90832.**

    b. If you spent 38 to 52 minutes providing psychotherapy, use code **90834**

    c. If you spent 53 to 89 minutes providing psychotherapy, use code **90837**

       i. If you spent longer than 89 minutes in the session, use **90837 + 99354**, the add-on code for extended time.

6.   If you provided an element of evaluation or management services for an **existing client**, you can choose the correct code either based on time spent providing care *or* on the complexity of your medical decision-making process. (The majority of E/M codes can be accurately selected based on time spent rendering care).

    a. Did you provide any psychotherapy services after rendering E/M care? If **yes**, choose the appropriate E/M code and then choose an add-on code to reflect time spent rendering psychotherapy:

       i. **E/M** + 30-minute psychotherapy session, use **+90833**

      ii. **E/M** + 45-minute psychotherapy session, use **+90836**

    iii. **E/M** + 60-minute psychotherapy session, use **+90838**

    iv. If using any of the psychotherapy add-on codes with an E/M code, then code **99354** for extended E/M time cannot be used.

    b. If no, select only one of the following codes based on time spent:

       i. If you spent 9 or fewer minutes rendering care, use **99211**

      ii. If you spent a total of 10-19 minutes rendering care, use **99212**

    iii. If you spent 20-29 minutes, use **99213**

    iv. If you spent 30-39 minutes, use **99214**

    v. If you spent 40-54 minutes, use **99215**

      vi. If you spent longer than 54 minutes rendering care, use **99215 + 99417**, the add-on code for prolonged E/M services.

7. When assessing a major change in the client's level of functioning, mental status, or the onset of a new symptoms for an existing client, you may be able to use a psychiatric diagnostic evaluation code *or* an E/M code. Consider:

    a. Has the client been billed for a **90791** or **90792** encounter during the past year?

      i. If yes, assess client's insurance coverage as most insurance payors will only cover one psychiatric diagnostic evaluation per year, while some may allow this code to be billed as often as every 6 months.

        1. If client is not eligible to be billed for a new psychiatric diagnostic evaluation, bill the E/M code that corresponds to the amount of time spent rendering services (**99211-99215**).

      ii. If no, and client is eligible to be billed for a psychiatric diagnostic exam, use code **90792** (unless it is a rare instance in which no medical services were rendered and code **90791** is more appropriate).

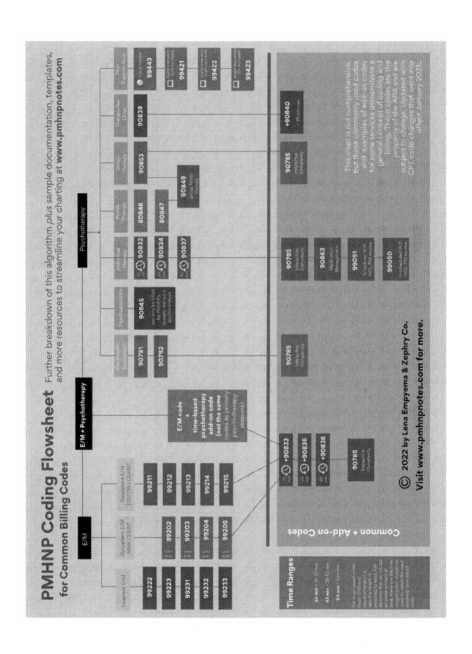

[5]

Using a Billing Code to Submit a Claim

Selecting the appropriate billing code for a client interaction is the first part of the billing process. Once the billing code is selected, you will need to ensure that your documentation fully supports the work you performed (thus justifying the code you are using to bill the insurance company), and that the proper paperwork is filled out accurately.

Introducing form CMS-1500.

While developed by the Centers for Medicare and Medicaid Services, CMS-1500 is used to submit claims for many private insurers as well. Of note, it may also be referred to as HCFA-1500.

The following image is a **sample** of CMS-1500. The image printed in this book should not be reproduced for the purpose of submitting a claim. Rather, providers must purchase an official CMS-1500 from a supplier due to unique ink color specification. If you do not yet have a supplier for CMS-1500, printers local to your office can be found using the hotline 1-866-512-1800 (U.S. Government Printing Office).

HEALTH INSURANCE CLAIM FORM

APPROVED BY NATIONAL UNIFORM CLAIM COMMITTEE (NUCC) 02/12

CARRIER

PATIENT AND INSURED INFORMATION

PHYSICIAN OR SUPPLIER INFORMATION

PICA

PICA

1. MEDICARE MEDICAID TRICARE CHAMPVA GROUP HEALTH PLAN FECA BLK LUNG OTHER | 1a. INSURED'S I.D. NUMBER (For Program in Item 1)

2. PATIENT'S NAME (Last Name, First Name, Middle Initial)
3. PATIENT'S BIRTH DATE SEX
4. INSURED'S NAME (Last Name, First Name, Middle Initial)

5. PATIENT'S ADDRESS (No., Street)
6. PATIENT RELATIONSHIP TO INSURED   Self Spouse Child Other
7. INSURED'S ADDRESS (No., Street)

CITY STATE
8. RESERVED FOR NUCC USE
CITY STATE

ZIP CODE TELEPHONE (Include Area Code)
ZIP CODE TELEPHONE (Include Area Code)

9. OTHER INSURED'S NAME (Last Name, First Name, Middle Initial)
10. IS PATIENT'S CONDITION RELATED TO:
11. INSURED'S POLICY GROUP OR FECA NUMBER

a. OTHER INSURED'S POLICY OR GROUP NUMBER
a. EMPLOYMENT? (Current or Previous) YES NO
a. INSURED'S DATE OF BIRTH SEX

b. RESERVED FOR NUCC USE
b. AUTO ACCIDENT? YES NO PLACE (State)
b. OTHER CLAIM ID (Designated by NUCC)

c. RESERVED FOR NUCC USE
c. OTHER ACCIDENT? YES NO
c. INSURANCE PLAN NAME OR PROGRAM NAME

d. INSURANCE PLAN NAME OR PROGRAM NAME
10d. CLAIM CODES (Designated by NUCC)
d. IS THERE ANOTHER HEALTH BENEFIT PLAN? YES NO If yes, complete items 9, 9a, and 9d.

READ BACK OF FORM BEFORE COMPLETING & SIGNING THIS FORM.

12. PATIENT'S OR AUTHORIZED PERSON'S SIGNATURE I authorize the release of any medical or other information necessary to process this claim. I also request payment of government benefits either to myself or to the party who accepts assignment below.

SIGNED _____ DATE _____

13. INSURED'S OR AUTHORIZED PERSON'S SIGNATURE I authorize payment of medical benefits to the undersigned physician or supplier for services described below.

SIGNED _____

14. DATE OF CURRENT ILLNESS, INJURY, or PREGNANCY (LMP) QUAL.
15. OTHER DATE QUAL.
16. DATES PATIENT UNABLE TO WORK IN CURRENT OCCUPATION FROM TO

17. NAME OF REFERRING PROVIDER OR OTHER SOURCE 17a. 17b. NPI
18. HOSPITALIZATION DATES RELATED TO CURRENT SERVICES FROM TO

19. ADDITIONAL CLAIM INFORMATION (Designated by NUCC)
20. OUTSIDE LAB? YES NO $ CHARGES

21. DIAGNOSIS OR NATURE OF ILLNESS OR INJURY Relate A-L to service line below (24E) ICD Ind.
A. B. C. D. E. F. G. H. I. J. K. L.
22. RESUBMISSION CODE ORIGINAL REF. NO.
23. PRIOR AUTHORIZATION NUMBER

24. A. DATES OF SERVICE From To		B. PLACE OF SERVICE	C. EMG	D. PROCEDURES, SERVICES, OR SUPPLIES (Explain Unusual Circumstances) CPT/HCPCS MODIFIER	E. DIAGNOSIS POINTER	F. $ CHARGES	G. DAYS OR UNITS	H. EPSDT Family Plan	I. ID QUAL.	J. RENDERING PROVIDER ID. #
MM DD YY MM DD YY									NPI	
1									NPI	
2									NPI	
3									NPI	
4									NPI	
5									NPI	
6									NPI	

25. FEDERAL TAX I.D. NUMBER SSN EIN
26. PATIENT'S ACCOUNT NO.
27. ACCEPT ASSIGNMENT? YES NO
28. TOTAL CHARGE $
29. AMOUNT PAID $ 0.00
30. Rsvd for NUCC Use

31. SIGNATURE OF PHYSICIAN OR SUPPLIER INCLUDING DEGREES OR CREDENTIALS (I certify that the statements on the reverse apply to this bill and are made a part thereof.)

SIGNED _____ DATE _____

32. SERVICE FACILITY LOCATION INFORMATION
33. BILLING PROVIDER INFO & PH #

NUCC Instruction Manual available at: www.nucc.org   PLEASE PRINT OR TYPE   APPROVED OMB-0938-1197 FORM 1500 (02-12)

Clear Form

60

Overview of Using CMS-1500

CMS-1500 is the standardized *health insurance claim form* used to submit claims to insurance payors. Just other discussions in this book have provided a basic overview of complex topics, this section, too, will provide basic knowledge of how to use the CMS-1500 form to submit insurance claims. Filling out this form in its entirety requires inputting specific information into the right boxes. CMS has published a 75-page guide detailing many of the nuances of the CMS-1500. It is available at:

https://www.cms.gov/regulations-and-guidance/guidance/manuals/downloads/clm104c26pdf.pdf

This form can be filled out electronically, or written by hand. If written by hand, all data must be clearly legible or you will risk a denial of your claim.

This chapter will discuss a specific section of the CMS-1500 which directly relates to billing codes. Billing codes and related confusion come into play in **section 24** of the CMS-1500.

Section 24 of CMS-1500

There are 10 components to section 24, labeled "24a" through "24j." Not all 10 boxes need to be filled out for every claim.

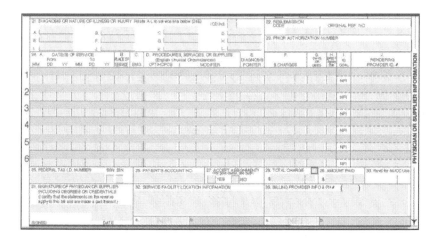

In section 24, there are 6 lines available for entering up to 6 CPT/HCPCS codes. Each of these 6 lines have a shaded component available for providing additional information.

Data for Sections 24a – 24j

(24a) Dates of service

For outpatient appointments, the start and end dates of service provided should be the same.

(24b) Place of service

A two-digit code. The full list is available on the CMS website at https://www.cms.gov/Medicare/Coding/place-of-service-codes/Place_of_Service_Code_Set.

Among the most common places of service for PMHNPs are:

10: *Telehealth.* To use this code, telecommunication services must be rendered while the client is located in their home.

11: *Office.* To use this code, services must be rendered in a clinic, which does not include hospitals, skilled nursing facilities, military treatment facilities, community health centers, or state or local public health clinics.

(24c) EMG (not a required field for Medicare reimbursement)

This section is only filled out if the services rendered were on an emergent or urgent basis. If applicable, 1 is used to denote emergency services and 2 is used to denote urgent services. If neither apply, this box is left blank.

(24d) CPT or HCPCS code

This is the place on the CMS-1500 where your billing codes are entered. The majority of this book discusses how to pinpoint the best billing code for any given service, and its technical application boils down to this single spot on a single form.

(also 24d) Modifier, if applicable

These codes indicate that there is a modification to the specific type of service described in the primary code submitted for billing purposes, but not a change significant enough to warrant the use of another code entirely. Depending on the modifier used, it may add information to a claim which does not result in a change in pricing, while other modifiers affect reimbursement rates.

Among the most common for PMHNPs include:

Telehealth service modifiers: 95, GQ, GT, G0 (zero)

Therapy modifiers: GN, GO, GP, KX, CO, CQ

(24e) Diagnosis pointer

The numbers for this section carry over from the diagnoses listed in section 21. In section 21 where the ICD-10 diagnoses are listed, each diagnosis is ranked in order of priority 1 indicates the primary diagnosis for service. Any additional diagnoses are ranked in descending order of prioritization. If there is only one diagnosis, enter 1.

(24f) Charges

In this section, enter the amount of money that you charge the general public for your services provided. Do not include a dollar sign.

There is a maximum rate for charges for each service. The maximum amount you are allowed to bill can be found using the lookup tool at www.cms.gov/medicare/physician-fee-schedule/search.

In the rare instance for PMHNPs that more than one unit of service is rendered, perform the multiplication of number of units *times* the amount you charge per unit and enter the total amount of charges in this box.

This section is most commonly used for billing multiple units of services such as mileage for an ambulance transport or another service that is easily multiplied. For outpatient PMHNPs, the most common codes are not subject to providing multiple units, and the charges can simply be entered as a single unit per billing code.

(24g) Days or Units (not a required field for Medicare reimbursement)

For instances like the above description where multiple units of service were rendered, box 24h to enter the number of units provided to the client. This is not a common occurrence for outpatient PMHNPs.

(24h) EPSDT (not a required field for Medicare reimbursement)

This refers to Early and Periodic Screening, Diagnosis, and Treatment, and is used when certain evaluations were provided. These types of screening and diagnoses vary among state-specific insurance plans and are not applicable in every state. For the purpose of brevity, this component will not be discussed in-depth.

Generally speaking, If an EPDST evaluation was performed, this box should be marked with an "X" and the appropriate E/M code must be used. Become familiar with the state-specific insurance plans that you accept to determine if this section is applicable to you in some situations.

(24i) ID Qualifier

Only used if the *billing provider* does not have an NPI number. If a licensed PMHNP is filling out this form, the PMHNP will have an NPI number and will not need to provide a non-NPI qualifier. This component may become applicable when using a billing service.

(24j) Rendering provider ID number

The PMHNP rendering the services will enter their NPI number in the non-shaded portion of this section. If using a billing service, the shaded portion will then be used to identify that billing provider.

[6]

Meeting Documentation Requirements

Overview of Clinical Documentation

The notes you use to record information in the clinical setting do more than provide a summary of what happened during any given appointment or interview. In addition to a complete and current depiction of the client's status, certain data must be included in every note to support your working diagnosis, justify your treatment plan, and ensure that payors have access to the information they need to process billing claims. These necessities complicate the documentation process and can leave PMHNPs guessing as to whether their charting practices are satisfactory.

While your specific documentation habits should satisfy the requirements of your place of employment, there are general guidelines for PMHNPs to follow regarding documentation.

Components Every Note Should Have:

- Patient identification
- Date of service rendered
- A "medically-appropriate" assessment
- Identification of the client's needs
- Treatment plan that realistically addresses client goals
- Demonstration of medical necessity
- Provider's legible signature and credentials

In mental health care, most clients are seen regularly, or at least scheduled for follow-up appointments following an initial treatment plan.

Minimum required notes to complete for each client as they progress through treatment:

- Initial assessment
- Progress notes written for each visit
- Discharge summary within five days of the last contact

Each piece of documentation should build upon previous notes so that there is an element of flow from one component to the next. The client's records should tell a complete story of their mental health care, beginning with the initial assessment and continuing logically through each progress note and treatment plan update.

Medicare and other payors require that the clock start and stop times of face-to-face counseling sessions appear in each note, not just the number of minutes that you spend with each client.

General Requirements of Documentation

Proving medical necessity to payors requires three components of documentation be met:

1. Adequate proof of diagnosis
2. Description of functional impairment
3. Clear plan for interventions to address impairments

To a third party reading your note, it should be clear why the client needs your services. Insurance payors will only approve care that is *needed*.

For example, if your proposed treatment plan includes helping a client develop a plan to ensure housing, medically necessitating your services as a clinician could be the inclusion of a statement such as, "the client's mental state and ongoing depression impairs her from following through to establish shelter."

Every note should clearly state the client's DSM-5 diagnosis, and highlight at least one functional impairment that the client has the potential to improve with the help of your services.

Example:

Diagnosis: Major Depressive Disorder

Functional impairment: Client reports hypersomnia which is affected her ability to concentrate at work and perform her job. Last month, the client lost her job, which was her only source of income. Unemployment has exacerbated client's feelings of hopelessness. Client is facing eviction and states that she has nowhere to go and no support system to help. The client's mental state and ongoing depression impairs her from following through to ensure shelter.

Treatment Plan: Refer client to the Emergency Rental Assistance program for help with rent during her time of hardship.

Establishing Medical Necessity

Through the entire care process, all services should be based upon *medical necessity* for the purposes of planning appropriate interventions and for accurate billing and coding.

Mental health documentation should include statements to support why the client needs your services. This data should also include a statement that the service you are providing will result in some level of *measurable improvement* in the client's condition or in maintenance of the client's health or mental health.

Payors use the medical record to determine the medical necessity. The medical record is the only source of information that payors have to evaluate for billing purposes. The payor must have access to clear and sufficient documentation for legal billing purposes.

The first step to establishing medical necessity occurs during the initial interview. During the initial interview, an assessment that captures both subjective and objective data helps generate an accurate diagnosis. Even when a firm diagnosis cannot be made during the first few meetings, a working diagnosis or differential diagnoses help guide follow-up meetings and drive the start of a treatment plan. The identification of a deficit in any area of the client's life and a treatment plan that addresses those deficits help define the medical necessity.

The client's reason for seeking treatment may or may not be sufficient to establish medical necessity. Progress notes should include your reasons for providing medically necessary care.

Specific to the common SOAP note format, medical necessity is established through the Assessment, while appropriate services are identified in the Plan.

The medical necessity should be established before mental health services are rendered to a client. When assessing objective and subjective data, specifying signs and symptoms that disrupt the client's functional ability to cope and perform standard activities of daily living provide the required documentation to establish medical necessity. Detailing the client's functional impairments in the Objective section help support the need for psychiatric services.

Diagnostic Criteria

In addition to clearly stating the diagnosis, your notes need to contain specific data that supports the diagnosis.

Proof of your diagnosis may appear in multiple parts of your notes.

- Within the PSFH, the patient's psychiatric history, family psychiatric history, and misuse or abuse of substances will detail the diagnosis.

- The review of systems will add more details to support your diagnosis.

- The subjective assessment data (including reported symptoms such as appetite and sleep quality) as well as the objective assessment data (including the MSE) will complete the picture of the diagnosis.

Functional Impairment

To prove that the client's diagnosis is affecting their functional abilities, there must be documentation of the functional impairment **or** documentation that there is a probability that the diagnosis will impact the client's functional abilities if left untreated. For children, evidence of impairment could also come in the form of a predicted impact on development if the psychiatric condition is left untreated.

This documentation will appear in your charting under the pertinent review of systems (if there is a physical manifestation). The bulk of the data will appear in the subjective and objective assessment data.

To satisfy the requirement of functional impairment criteria, the mental disorder that fits the diagnostic criteria should be documented as causing one of the following:

1. A significant impairment in an activity of daily living
2. The probability that an important area of functioning will deteriorate without treatment
3. *(For children)* the probability that the child will not develop appropriately without treatment

Functional areas that may be affected include:

- Feelings, mood, or affect
- Thinking
- Interpersonal or familial relationships
- Social isolation

- Work performance
- Socio-legal conduct
- Self-care or activities of daily living

The interventions will appear in the assessment portion of the SOAP note because this section contains the treatment options for the client. The bulk of this data will appear under the "plan" in the form of medication changes, referrals, and disposition. Proof of how your proposed interventions will improve the client's functional impairments can be as simple as adding a short explanation to the end of the sentence.

Examples:

Client to begin lamotrigine **to stabilize her mood.**

Client to continue weekly therapy sessions **to assist him in processing emotions related to his son's death.**

Intervention Criteria

The intervention-related criteria should meet all of the following:

1. Proposed interventions should focus on addressing the conditions identified in the impairment criteria
2. Proposed interventions should benefit the client by significantly diminishing the impairment
   - (or) the proposed interventions should prevent probable deterioration in an important area of functioning
3. The diagnosed condition would not be responsive to physical health care or standard medical interventions, thus necessitating psychiatric care

Interventions that can be provided to alleviate the problem. Shows how it can be fixed. Explain how your interventions can help.

While you can't guarantee anything or foresee the future or even predict a timeline: based on history and current symptoms, take an educated guess for how interventions could help and how long it could take.

If you don't meet the timeline, you can adjust at the end of the projected timeline. Use the medical necessity language to

Common Documentation Questions

"How long should the note be for any given appointment?"

There is no specific designated length in terms of pages or words that a note should satisfy. Rather, the note should simply tell a complete story of the encounter with the client.

"How do I decide which ICD-10 codes to include?"

There are more than 70,000 available ICD-10 codes at the time of publishing. These codes are periodically updated. Online search sites that can facilitate looking up applicable codes quickly and easily. One of the best is available for free at:

https://www.icd10data.com/

"If there is no change in patient status, can I copy the majority of the note from the last visit?"

Portions of previous narratives should not be copied from previous notes and pasted into new notes without significant updating and/or editing to ensure that the information you document is as accurate, thorough, and up-to-date as possible.

The safest way to save time when writing notes is to use a template which auto-populates the beginning of sentences and leaves open-ended space to customize each sentence in the note for the specific patient on the day of the appointment. This template format prevents copying and pasting whole sentences, which could increase the chances of raising a flag for potential fraud. The templates at www.pmhnpnotes.com that I drafted for my on-demand note assistance course are written in this way to allow for fast, easy customization and point-click pasting into the EMR.

Wording notes too similarly could raise alarms for payors and other auditors that a potential duplication of services may have occurred. In some states and situations, inaccurate or outdated information is considered fraudulent, an offense which can affect not only reimbursement for services rendered but also professional licensure.

"Who reads the notes I write?"

New laws originally scheduled to take effect in 2020 and then delayed until 2021 make the majority of the notes you write as a PMHNP available to your clients to read in full.

What does this change?

Theoretically, the increased accessibility to notes should not change the way you document nor the content of your notes. Even prior to these new laws taking place, there was an omnipresent possibility that any client could obtain access to his or her medical records through a medical records office. In practice, however, understanding that your audience has likely increased is another reason to ensure that your notes are as thorough and accurate as possible, and that the entirety of their content is worded in a clear, professional tone that cannot be misconstrued.

Common Mistakes in Mental Health Notes

To better comprehend how to write a comprehensive and satisfactory note, it is easiest to first understand the most common mistakes that PMHNPs make in documentation.

- **Choosing the wrong billing code**
- **Documentation does not support diagnosis**
- Incomplete documentation of therapy services specific to time, goals, treatment plan and status
- Initial assessments not including treatment plan
- Incomplete E&M services missing pertinent history,
- Missing components of the Mental Status Exam
- Omitting negative findings (charting by exception)
- Missing response to medication and education
- Progress notes not tied to care plans in a meaningful way
- No documentation of skilled interventions provided
- No documentation of clinical progress (symptom resolution, etc.)
- Recording wrong amount of time spent with patient

The first two items topping the list of common mistakes in documentation are the wrong billing code and/or documentation failing to support the diagnosis. These factors are both strongly tied to clinical notes.

If one or more insurance claims are denied due to these reasons, some providers can conclude that their notes are not long enough. The process of documentation then becomes even more stressful as providers add length to notes in hopes of capturing all necessary data.

However, the actual problem usually is not that the note is too *short*, but that the *wrong data* is included. Most PMHNP notes are not lacking in length, just lacking the specific data that should be included for a particular billing code.

For example, failing to include the symptoms that the client exhibited to support your diagnosis, or not including the review of recent blood tests that you reviewed that supported the E/M code you billed can create issues with insurance reimbursement.

Formatting Mental Health Notes

There is no single acceptable format for your clinical notes, leaving room for you to organize them in the way that works best for you.

The most popular formats for notes include:

- SOAP
- BIRP
- DAP
- DRAP
- Unstructured notes

SOAP is a preferred format for many providers for medical-centered encounters. "**SOAP**" in regards to mental health notes refers to a comprehensive format for capturing information. SOAP notes are one of the most common formats for an initial intake assessment or initial client interview. This format is also used for many follow-up assessments and psychotherapy appointments to ensure that pertinent data is recorded.

BIRP which stands for Behavior, Intervention, Response, and Plan. BIRP works well for documenting progress notes for existing clients. If you prefer the BIRP format, there is no reason BIRP notes cannot be written for your client encounters as long as all pertinent information is satisfactorily captured.

The **DAP** format structures notes in the order of Data, Assessment, and Plan.

Similarly, **DRAP** refers to Data, Reaction, Assessment, and Plan.

Because the SOAP format has the potential to capture all pertinent information, whether for an initial interview or for a more abbreviated follow-up meeting and can be easily modified for length, SOAP is the format most prominently presented in this particular resource.

Using SOAP to capture Sufficient Data for Billing and Coding

As aforementioned, there are multiple acceptable formats for your mental health notes. **SOAP** notes are one of the more popular formats, but the **DAP** format is used commonly as well. Another option is the **BIRP.**

As my format of choice is the SOAP note, I created a graphic to display where the pertinent data should fit into the SOAP:

How the **SOAP format** helps PMHNPs capture sufficient data for billing & coding purposes:

S

Client's symptoms that prove the diagnosis

Client's account of functional impairment

O

Observations of client's functional impairment

Signs and outward manifestations that prove the diagnosis

A

Interventions to address functional impairment

Progress towards goals to support medical necessity

P

Implementation of interventions to help client work towards goals

Proposed timeline of interventions to address functional impairments

ZEPHRY CO

SOAP Notes for Mental Health Care

SOAP: Subjective, Objective, Assessment, Plan

SOAP notes can be a mix of bullet points and narrative text, though the bulk of most SOAP notes is written in narrative form to ensure that a complete story is told.

Information gathered during face-to-face interviews makes up the Subjective and Objective sections of the SOAP. You as the clinician should guide the client and any other supporting members through the interview in a way that facilitates gathering as much data as possible for the Subjective portion of the note while also collecting observations that you will detail in the Objective portion of the note.

How Psychiatric SOAP Notes Differ from Other Specialties

For PMHNPs transitioning to a mental health care role from an area with greater emphasis on medical care, documenting satisfactory SOAP notes that provide sufficient information for follow-up care and billing purposes can be confusing. However, the concept of the SOAP note is the same with a focus on different aspects of the assessment and more significant subjective data collection from the face-to-face interview.

With fewer laboratory tests that capture quantitative data, the objective portion of the SOAP note can be leaner than SOAP notes for NPs in other specialties.

In mental health care, there is less emphasis on medical testing and the review of systems. While both medical testing and a pertinent review of systems can be included in a mental health SOAP note whenever applicable, the bulk of the data is the subjective section which captures the client's symptoms, complaints, and goals, and the objective signs and physical manifestations that you as the clinician will observe and report during the interview.

<u>S</u>: Subjective Data

The first step of a client interview is to gather all the information that the client has to share about their own symptoms, in their own words. Data should include a history of the present illness as well as the current status of symptoms, and the client's goals for their treatment. You will gather this data during the initial interview

Subjective data should be recorded using direct quotes from the client whenever possible rather than paraphrasing to capture the most insight. Contributions from family members or other supporting members present for the interview can also be included using quotes.

This portion of the patient's record serves as the basis for the treatment plan and lays the foundation for the rest of the notes, so collecting enough quality subjective information is crucial.

The following lists of data that should appear in the "S" portion of the psychiatric SOAP notes are comprehensive. Every component of data may not apply to every client, but any data pertinent to differential diagnoses should be detailed in the medical record.

History of Present Illness (HPI) as Reported by Client:

- Medical diagnoses
- Hospitalizations (medical and psychiatric)
- Previous outpatient or residential programs
- Previous individual or group psychotherapy
- Past trauma
- Medical or surgical procedures
- Previous self-injurious behaviors
- SI/SA
- HA

Family History:

- Suicides and homicides in family
- Suicide or homicide attempts in family
- Long-term institutional treatment of family

Subjective Data to Obtain During Interview:

- Client's chief complaint
- Names and relationships of others present for the interview
- Basic demographic information
- Gender, gender expression, and preferred pronouns
- Appetite
- Sleep quality
- Level of physical activity

- Current and past medications used to manage reported symptoms and existing diagnoses
- Client's perceived efficacy of medications
- Client's compliance with medication regimen
- Other medications, including vitamins and daily supplements
- Pertinent recent lab results

Social History:

- Highest level of education
- Occupation, if applicable, and current employment status
- Living situation
- Support system
- Sexual activity
- Contraceptive practices (to include birth control, condoms, etc.)
- Use of substances such as alcohol and recreational drugs
- Smoking status

What is *not appropriate* to include in this portion of the SOAP note?

- Information that the client requests be kept confidential as long as the data doesn't violate the duty to protect
- Confidential HIV status

- Self-reported alcohol misuse or illegal use of illicit substances if client does not agree to disclosure

Client's Goals for Treatment

- Must be measurable or quantifiable
- Must be stated in terms of the reported or observed impairment
- Should relate to impaired aspects of functional areas of life
  - Living situation, activities of daily living, school, work, social support system, legal, physical health, psychiatric health, and/or substance use or misuse
- Should include opportunities for incremental achievements
- Should be time-limited achievable in a reasonable timeframe
- Should be clearly stated so that the client can effectively work towards achievement

O: Objective Data

The second section of the psychiatric SOAP note should detail objective facts and data from an impartial point of view. Detailed, factual observations about the patient and physical manifestations of conditions are important to help round out the client's medical record. The Objective section should also include a thorough Mental Status Exam and risk assessment.

The focus of the objective portion of the note should build upon what you learned during the subjective portion of the interview. For example, if a client reported feeling symptoms of nervousness and overwhelming worry during the subjective portion of the interview, you as the practitioner should observe any physical manifestations of anxiety, such as trembling hands, rapid speech, or clenching the jaw. Similarly, if a client reports feeling anxious but exhibits a relaxed posture with no outward physical manifestations of the reported symptoms, the negative observations should also be included in this section.

Performing a Risk Assessment:

- "Do you feel safe?"
- "Do you have any thoughts or plans to harm yourself?"
- "Do you have any thoughts or plans to harm someone else?"
- (If yes to either of the previous two questions) "Do you intend to follow through on those plans?"
- "Has anything happened recently to cause these thoughts or plans?"

Pertinent Review of Systems:

- Much less detailed than a medical SOAP note
- If no pertinent assessment findings, charting "unremarkable, noncontributory, insignificant, or negative" for the ROS is acceptable

Objective Data Should Include:

- Pertinent review of systems (ROS)
- Description of client's physical appearance
- Vital signs, lab results, and test results as transcribed from medical records or ordered by you
- Abnormal physical manifestations such as tremors or tics
- Observations of signs that could relate to a differential diagnosis or the rule-out of a differential diagnosis

What is *not appropriate* to include in this portion of the SOAP note?

- Urine drug screen results (unless have member consent)
- Observations of behavior of family members or other member collaterals in therapy sessions
- Reports made as a mandatory reporter for suspicion of child or elder abuse

<u>A</u>: Assessment Data

The Assessment portion of the note should establish medical necessity. Using the information gathered in the Subjective and Objective sections of the SOAP note, you will interpret the data and document your impressions in the Assessment section. The Assessment section of the first note you write for a client may or may not provide a diagnosis. If the assessment findings are straightforward enough for you to provide a clear diagnosis, it should be documented in this section. Otherwise, you should continue to explore differential diagnoses in this section.

For SOAP notes written after the first visit, the Assessment section should also include a narrative of how the client is progressing towards his or her treatment goals and whether improvements noted in previous sessions are being maintained.

Assessment Should Include:

- DSM-5 diagnoses
- Differential psychiatric diagnoses
- Concurrent medical diagnoses
- Corresponding ICD-10 codes
- Treatment options
- Client input regarding treatment options
- Obstacles to successful treatment

- Evaluation of client safety
- Client needs for social services

(After the first visit) Assessment Should Include:

- Progress towards goal achievement
- Applicable changes in degree of risk

What is *not appropriate* to include in this portion of the SOAP note?

- Your assessment of compliance with court-ordered treatments
- evaluation of the status of client's relationships
- Evaluation of the client's parenting skills
- Prognosis for the likelihood the client with achieve sobriety from drugs and/or alcohol

P: Plan

Using the diagnoses established in the assessment, the plan should detail actionable items and the proposed course of treatment.

For clients receiving treatment for multiple conditions, there should be a separate plan for each condition. The diagnoses addressed can be the conclusions that you established based on interview findings, or could be based on diagnoses that other clinicians provided. The information in this section should address all of the deficits that you described in the Assessment.

During every visit, the plan should be reevaluated and any adjustments should be made as necessary.

Plan should include:

- Treatment that the client received today
- Rationale for providing that treatment
- Client's immediate response to treatment
- Plan for follow-up such as when the client will return for additional treatment
- Instructions given to the client
- Outcome measures for problems
- Medications, dosing, and titrations (new or changes)
- Lab work to order or reevaluate
- Referrals to psychiatric or medical providers
- Referrals to social or community services
- Therapy recommendations
- Holistic and complementary options to explore
- Education provided to client
- Instructions provided to client
- The rationale for your decisions
- When to schedule next appointment for client

What is *not appropriate* to include in this portion of the SOAP note?

- Plans for legally mandated reporting (e.g., child abuse, elder abuse)
- Information about referrals of family members or other member collaterals for individual or family treatment service

Sample statements for Plan:

- "Clinician will support client to express unresolved grief to reduce symptoms of depression in biweekly individual sessions for the next six months."
- "Over the next six months, clinician will meet with the client or initiate a telehealth appointment two to three times per week to teach, model, and implement social and adult living skills necessary to help maintain housing."
- "Clinician to provide medication management two to six times per three-month period to decrease anxiety."
- "Plan is to collaborate with treatment team, including psychiatrist, psychotherapist, and community support workers a minimum of three times per month to provide continuity of care."

[7]

Sample Notes for Specific Billing Codes

Psychiatric Diagnostic Evaluation

Documentation must include:

- Complete medical history
- Complete psychiatric history
- Complete social history
- Complete family history
- Initial diagnosis
- Evaluation of client's ability and capacity to respond to treatments rendered
- Plan of treatment

90792 Note Example

The documentation for 90791 and 90792 is similar, with the exception of the medical service rendered in 90792. Because PMHNPs are licensed medical professionals, it is common to provide a medical service in a psychiatric diagnostic evaluation.

For visits in which no medical service is provided, your documentation will be the same as the note below except there will be no medical services (a physical exam or prescription, for example) documented.

Example on following page:

Date of service: January 1, 20XX

I spent 62 minutes meeting with the client today to perform a psychiatric diagnostic evaluation. Client is seeking care for "feeling a lot more anxious lately" to the extent that her symptoms are affecting her quality of sleep and ability to function at work.

The client provided a complete medical history and previous psychiatric history, which I reviewed in totality.

Client states she has "always been a worrier" but for the past four months, she feels racing thoughts throughout the day and fixates on "little things that wouldn't have bothered her before." Client cannot recall a specific precipitating event that caused the change in her level of worry. Client works full-time as a bank teller and has two children living at home who are both high school students. Client is heterosexual, married to a male, and denies recent changes in the status of her relationship with her spouse.

Client states her appetite has been normal. Sleep quality has been poor. Client does not take medications to help her sleep. States she has "tried Unisom and Benadryl years ago, but they make me feel hungover in the mornings." Client drinks an estimated three cups of coffee per day. Drinks beer "mostly on the weekends." States she never drinks more than four beers per day.

Client's medical history is significant for ulcerative colitis, obesity, and hypertension. Client's blood pressure is well controlled on lisinopril 10 mg taken daily. Client has taken this medication for an estimated four years. Client receives Remicade infusions every eight weeks to control ulcerative colitis symptoms. Client has been on this medication for two years with no adverse effects and states UC symptoms are well controlled with current treatment. Client reports having been overweight for the majority of her adult life. Current BMI is 32. Client states she has little time to exercise or meal plan with the demands of her work and family obligations.

In addition to prescription lisinopril and Remicade, client reports taking two OTC herbal ashwagandha capsules daily. Client states she follows the directions on the bottle but cannot remember the dose of each capsule. Client began taking ashwagandha three months ago hoping it would help manage her feelings of anxiety. Client reports noticing no improvement in her symptoms since taking ashwagandha.

Family medical history positive for heart disease (mother, maternal grandmother) and lung cancer (paternal grandfather).

Client has no previous psychiatric history. Client has not previously sought treatment her symptoms of anxiety.

I evaluated the client's mental status. Client is alert and fully oriented with adequate insight and judgement. Client sits on the edge of the chair for session and fidgets with hands for duration of visit. At times, speech is rapid. Appearance and behavior are appropriate. Client convincingly denies thoughts of self-harm, suicide, and homicide.

The working diagnosis is generalized anxiety disorder (F41.1).

The initial plan of treatment includes weekly talk

therapy sessions to occur for 12 weeks. Discussed journaling with client and suggested that client spend 10-15 daily writing her symptoms in a journal as well as stressors she experiences in preparation for first session, which is scheduled for Tuesday at 9:00. Provided education on the impact of caffeine on symptoms of anxiety and suggested that client try decaffeinated coffee as part of her morning routine this week.

Considering client's history, familial support system, and motivation, prognosis is good. The client demonstrated the ability to respond positively to this plan of treatment and, with adherence to chosen interventions, should demonstrate progress towards her goals.

Lena Empyema
Lena Empyema, MSN, PMH-NP

Outpatient E/M

New Client E/M Example

Date of service: January 1, 20XX

Client is new to this practice and seeking care for depressive symptoms. Client states, "I have been tired and not really feeling myself." Client initially sought treatment with primary care physician for chronic fatigue and weight gain of 20 pounds over the last 6 months. PCP ruled out common medical causes of chronic fatigue and weight gain and referred client to mental health care for suspected depression.

I spent 35 minutes providing care for this client, including time spent reviewing labs ordered by PCP. [See results in Client History in EMR]. Discussed recent life changes extensively with client as well as client's goals for treatment, to include "feeling back to normal." I arranged for follow-up psychotherapy to begin weekly pending client's insurance approval.

The client completed a New Client Intake Form [see complete form in EMR] and self-reported the following components, which I reviewed and discussed with the client.

- Chief complaint
- Current symptoms
- History of present illness
- Medication reconciliation
- Medical/surgical history
- Psychiatric history
- Social history and lifestyle
- Family history
- Use of alcohol and illicit substances
- Suicide self-assessment

Significant findings among these components include:

- Symptoms of tiredness and weight gain congruent with a diagnosis of depression.
- No previous psychiatric diagnoses.
- Family history includes a mother diagnosed with depression x 20 years.

I performed a review of systems. See EMR for client's vital signs, height, and weight. All findings were negative with the exception of the following findings:

- BMI > 30. Client states she diets "on and off."

Working diagnosis: Depression. Will update as more information becomes available.

Initial treatment plan: Weekly individual talk therapy. Client open to trialing antidepressant medication after further evaluation.

Lena Empyema
Lena Empyema, MSN, PMH-NP

Discussion of this note:

- Clock start and stop times are no longer required to satisfy billing requirements. Instead, I specified the total number of minutes I spent on this visit (35 minutes). As of the 2021 changes to CPT codes, E/M codes can be selected based on time. On that basis, a 35-minute E/M visit for a new client should be billed as **99203.**
- In two places, I referred to more thorough documentation that is available in the EMR. I do not need to "double document" this data, and can instead refer the reviewer to another part of the official medical record to find details. Rather than typing the negative findings, I highlighted only the positive findings. The negative data (such as no former surgical history, no current use of alcohol or illicit substances, etc.) is still documented in the record and reviewed by the provider.
- I included the working diagnosis and the initial treatment plan, as well as the client's goal to "feel normal," stated in her own words. The chief complaint is also stated early in the note in the client's own words.
- This same format with similar content can be used for other E/M codes for new clients and adjusted based on time spent in the visit or based on the level of medical decision-making, if not congruent with time spent.
- If this visit also included psychotherapy, I could still bill as 99203 for the E/M component, then use an add-on code for psychotherapy based on how long the psychotherapy session lasted:
    - 90833 (16-37 minutes of psychotherapy)
    - 90836 (38-52 minutes of psychotherapy)
    - 90838 (53+ minutes of psychotherapy)

Established Client E/M Example

Date of service: January 1, 20XX

This client is well-known to this practice where he receives care for attention deficit disorder. As part of this visit, I reviewed previously reported information on the Client Intake forms (see EMR). No updates necessary with the exception of:

- Client had his wisdom teeth surgically removed since last visit. No complications, and no new prescriptions.

I spent 22 minutes providing care for this client, including time spent discussing client's performance in school since last visit and sleep habits. Client reported passing grades in all subjects and feels that he is progressing towards his goals of improving academic performance enough to graduate at the end of the spring semester. Client has also started a new part-time working ten hours per week at a carwash. Client does not feel that the job is affecting his academic performance, and does feel that his current dosage of methylphenidate is sufficient to continue progressing in school and concentrating at work. No adjustments to prescription will be made at this time.

I performed a review of systems. See EMR for client's vital signs, height, and weight. All findings were negative.

Scheduled follow-up appointment for three months from now to ensure that client continues to progress towards goals.

Lena Empyema
Lena Empyema, MSN, PMH-NP

Discussion of this note:

- o The time ranges corresponding to E/M codes for established clients are different than the time ranges for new clients. I spent 22 minutes with this client, which correlates to a CPT code of **99213**.
- o The narrative regarding the extent of discussion with the client is perhaps lengthier than necessary. A more abbreviated narrative should suffice to meet the documentation requirements for this particular visit.

"I still feel overwhelmed by documentation requirements."

If this sounds like you, I have more resources to share.

I created www.PMHNPNotes.com to provide even more resources for PMHNPs and PMHNP students.

More than just bland educational content, my **Quick & Comprehensive PMHNP Note** e-course is also a database of downloads such as intake forms and blank assessment and screening tools to make documentation the easiest part of your job (even if it's your least favorite task right now!).

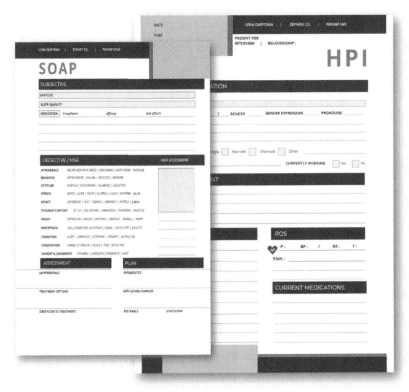

Providers asked. I listened.

I also created a unique and aesthetically pleasing two-page data collection form to minimize the amount of writing you need to do during any given session. No need to decipher pages of scribbles at the end of a long day or week.

This document is available as a full-color download at www.pmhnpnotes.com, or as a perfect-bound paperback on Amazon with free shipping for Prime members!

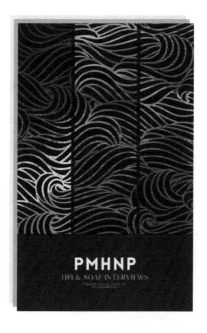

This book is on Amazon. Find PMHNP HPI & SOAP Interview by Lena Empyema on Amazon.

References

American Psychiatric Association. *Diagnostic and Statistical Manual of Mental Disorders, Fifth Edition (DSM-5).* 2013.

Arcangelo, V.P. & Peterson, A.M. (2006). Pharmacotherapeutics for advanced practice: A
practical approach (2nd ed.). Philadelphia: Lippincott Williams & Wilkins.

Beck, David E, and David A Margolin. "Physician coding and reimbursement." *The Ochsner journal* vol. 7,1 (2007): 8-15.

Bedard, N. A., Carender, C. N., DeMik, D. E., Browne, J. A., Schwarzkopf, R., & Callaghan, J. J. (2021). The Impact of Transitioning From International Classification of Diseases, Ninth Revision to International Classification of Diseases, Tenth Revision on Reported Complication Rates Following Primary Total Knee Arthroplasty. *The Journal of Arthroplasty, 36*(5), 1617-1620.

Bickley, L. S. (2009). Bates' pocket guide to physical examination and history taking (6th ed.). Philadelphia: Lippincott Williams & Wilkins.

Birch, K., Ling, A., & Phoenix, B. (2021). Psychiatric nurse practitioners as leaders in behavioral health integration. *The Journal for Nurse Practitioners, 17*(1), 112-115.

Brown, J. D., Urato, C., & Ogbuefi, P. (2021). Uptake of Medicare behavioral health integration billing codes in 2017 and 2018. *Journal of General Internal Medicine, 36*(2), 564-566.

Church, S. L., Solis, E., & Moore, K. J. (2021). The 2021 Medicare Payment and CPT Coding Update. *Family Practice Management, 28*(1).

Dissociative Experiences Scale - II. (Dec 08, 2021). Traumadissociation.com. Retrieved Dec 8, 2021 from http://traumadissociation.com/des. Try it yourself: http://traumadissociation.com/des

Domino, F. J. (Eds.). (2010). The 5-minute clinical consult. Philadelphia: Lippincott Williams & Wilkins.

Elsevier. (2021). *Buck's 2021 HCPCS Level II-E-Book*. Saunders.

First MB, Williams JBW, Karg RS, Spitzer RL: Structured Clinical Interview
for DSM-5 Disorders, Clinician Version (SCID-5-CV). Arlington,
VA, American Psychiatric Association, 2016:
https://www.appi.org/products/structured-clinical-interview-
for-dsm-5-scid-
5#:~:text=About%20the%20SCID%2D5,5%20classification%20and
%20diagnostic%20criteria

Harsora P, Kessmann J. Nonpharmacologic management of chronic
insomnia. Am Fam Physician. 2009 Jan 15;79(2):125-30.

Hovey, B. A. (2021). Telemedicine Billing and Coding. In *Telemedicine in
Orthopedic Surgery and Sports Medicine* (pp. 29-41). Springer, Cham.

Kameg, B. N., & Kameg, K. (2021). An Update on Billing and Coding for
the Psychiatric–Mental Health Nurse Practitioner. *Journal of
Psychosocial Nursing and Mental Health Services*, 1-3.

Kumari S, Malik M, Florival C, Manalai P, Sonje S. An Assessment of Five
(PANSS, SAPS, SANS, NSA-16, CGI-SCH) commonly used
Symptoms Rating Scales in Schizophrenia and Comparison to
Newer Scales (CAINS, BNSS). J Addict Res Ther. 2017;8(3):324.
doi:10.4172/2155-6105.1000324.

McNeese, K. A. (2021). Utilization and Documentation of Hospital
Admission Depression Screening: A Quality Improvement Project.

Morgenthaler T, Kramer M, Alessi C, Friedman L, Boehlecke B, Brown T,
Coleman J, Kapur V, Lee-Chiong T, Owens J, Pancer J, Swick T;
American Academy of Sleep Medicine. Practice parameters for the
psychological and behavioral treatment of insomnia: an update.
An american academy of sleep medicine report. Sleep. 2006
Nov;29(11):1415-9.

Morin CM, Vallières A, Guay B, Ivers H, Savard J, Mérette C, Bastien C,
Baillargeon L. Cognitive behavioral therapy, singly and combined
with medication, for persistent insomnia: a randomized controlled
trial. JAMA. 2009 May 20;301(19):2005-15.

Rifkin A. Extrapyramidal side effects: a historical perspective. *J Clin
Psychiatry*. 1987 Sep;48(Suppl):3–6. [PubMed].

Riley M, Ahmed S, Locke A. Common Questions About Oppositional
Defiant Disorder. Am Fam Physician. 2016 Apr 1;93(7):586-91.
PMID: 27035043.

Schutte-Rodin S, Broch L, Buysse D, Dorsey C, Sateia M. Clinical guideline
for the evaluation and management of chronic insomnia in adults.
J Clin Sleep Med. 2008 Oct 15;4(5):487-504.

Steiner H, Remsing L; Work Group on Quality Issues. Practice parameter
for the assessment and treatment of children and adolescents with
oppositional defiant disorder. J Am Acad Child Adolesc
Psychiatry. 2007 Jan;46(1):126-141. doi:
10.1097/01.chi.0000246060.62706.af. PMID: 17195736

Made in the USA
Columbia, SC
20 December 2024

50246035R10063